How to Receive Healing and Bring Healing to Others

Volume 2
in the Healing Series

By Prince Handley

University of Excellence Press

Copyright © 2012 Prince Handley
All Rights Reserved.

UNIVERSITY OF EXCELLENCE PRESS
Los Angeles ◾ London ◾ Tel Aviv

ISBN-13: 978-0692334232
ISBN-10: 0692334238

Printed in the U.S.A.

Second Edition

TABLE OF CONTENTS

INTRODUCTION

My goal is to define the parameters in which **you can be healed** scripturally and live in health ... and then **you can help others** do the same!

Physical and mental healing belong to you as much as spiritual healing. In this book you will learn HOW to obtain total healing through various tools with specific instructions.

How to use the **healing tools of God** with examples are included.

Key Points:

> ■ The LORD's healing nature never changes.

> ■ It is God's will to heal you!

> ■ Know that healing belongs to you because God has given you specific TOOLS of healing!

Your friend,
Prince Handley

How to Receive Healing and Bring Healing to Others

Volume 2
in the Healing Series

God's Tools for Healing You

Yeshua fulfilled what Isaiah the prophet said **750 years before** in Isaiah Chapter 53:

> He bore **our** sicknesses and diseases.
> He carried away **our** pains.
> With his stripes **WE ARE HEALED**.

Yeshua's body and mind took punishment for **us**...his blood paid for **our** sins. His body was beaten, wounded, and bruised (even before he was crucified), and then he was nailed to the wooden cross...FOR **OUR** HEALING: spiritual, physical, and mental!

Oppression–both mental and physical–are included in Yeshua's work for **us**. Messiah was driven; he was abased and looked down upon. Isaiah 53:7 says, **"He was oppressed and he was afflicted..."** In Isaiah 53:4, where it reads, **" ...he carried our 'pains'..."**, the literal Hebrew meaning is **"acute pain; intense suffering: MENTAL or PHYSICAL."** What Yesua did FOR you, you don't have to do!

Yeshua healed the separation between G-d and man through his work FOR US, and therefore ended Satan's dominion over ALL who would trust in Messiah! *"For this purpose the Son of God was manifested, that he might DESTROY the works of the devil."* (1 John 3:8)

Yeshua (Jesus, the Messiah) **"carried"** sickness, sin, disease, poverty, and oppression– the works of the devil (Satan) – FOR YOU. Now you don't have to carry them any longer. They do NOT belong to the believer in Messiah Yeshua! WHAT YESHUA DID FOR YOU ... YOU DON'T HAVE TO DO!

Now that you know that physical and mental healing belong to the believer in Messiah Jesus

-- as much as spiritual healing – you need to know how to obtain it: **How to be healed!** There are several tools, or methods, **to obtain AND to minister** Messiah's healing power. They are listed below:

- THE WORD OF GOD
- LAYING ON OF HANDS
- HOLY COMMUNION
- ANOINTING WITH OIL
- PRAYER & PROPER MENTAL ATTITUDE

First, I'm going to teach you how to be healed through **the Word of God**.

THE WORD OF GOD

The Holy Bible says, *"He sent his word, and healed them, and delivered them from their destructions."* (Psalm 107:20.) God's Word heals: God's nature is healing, and he has given LIFE to his Word. You can be healed by knowing what God promises in his Word concerning healing. Find the promises G-d has made you in the Holy Bible for healing and for health, and then appropriate one or more of these promises for yourself.

Speak the promises of God to yourself (or to others). Your faith will rise as you do. *"So then faith comes by hearing, and hearing by the Word of God."* (Romans 10:17) As you confess (or speak aloud) the promises of God, your healing

7

will come. Don't worry if you don't see it as soon as you think you should…it has to happen!

Yeshua taught that what you speak will come to pass if you believe it in your heart (Mark 11:23). Don't talk sickness, or doubt, or unbelief anymore…start talking healing, faith, and belief…based upon what your Father God has promised you! Hearing and meditating upon the Word of God produce healing, also. I have known people to be healed of conditions they have had for years by HEARING God's Word while I was preaching (both in worship services indoors and preaching outdoors).

"And they went forth, and preached everywhere, the Lord working with them, and confirming the word with signs following." (Mark 16:20)

Meditating (thinking deeply or fixing attention) upon God's Word brings life and health, also. Proverbs 4:20-22 tells us:

"My son, attend to my words; incline [or, direct] your ear unto my sayings. Let them not depart from your eyes; keep them in the middle of your heart. For they are LIFE unto those that find them, and HEALTH to all their flesh."

HEALING BY ATTENDING
TO THE WORD OF GOD

In the Proverbs we are instructed as follows:

*"My son, **attend** to my words. Turn your **ear** to my sayings. Let them not depart from your **eyes**. Keep them in the midst of your **heart**. For they are **life** to those who find them, And **health** to their whole body."* Proverbs 4:20-22.

To **attend** means: **to be present, to focus, to think about**. This passage shows us **HOW to attend to the Words of God**. To attend to His Word – and His PROMISES – of healing:

> We must have an **attentive ear**.
> We must have a **steady and fixed look**.
> We must have a **receptive heart**.

There are so many promises in the word of God that pertain to divine healing and health. We have covered many of them in *How to be Healed and Live in Divine Health* (Volume 1 in the e-Book HEALING series).

Also, for a complete resource on Health and Healing, go here: *Health and Healing Complete Guide to Wholeness.* It is available in both Kindle and paperback book formats.

However, if you are in need of healing NOW, it is important to attend to these promises by:

An **attentive ear**
A **steady and fixed look,** and
A **receptive heart**.

Listen to the promises. If you do not have access to some means of hearing via a recorded message, then just **speak the promises aloud to yourself**. I do this every day. I have been on Planet Earth a long time. The doctor I had for years used to tell me, "God heals and doctors get the credit." The last time I had an Annual Physical from him he asked me, "Do you want to come back in one or two years?"

It is good to feel healthy. And, **health** is not only a **gift** from God, but a **promise** from God. **Look at the promises**. Read them and look closely at them. **Focus on them** by meditating upon them: through your eyes AND in your mind. This way you will be able to **SEE** them at any time on the screen of your mind (if not verbatim, at least the content of the promises). They are your life blood–literally–when you need healing. That is **WHY** God has given them to you.

Receive the promises. Think about the **gift** which God is offering you. **A gift has to be received**. Realize that God loves you so much that He has provided healing for you through His Son: Yeshua ha Mashiach (Jesus the Messiah). Healing ... and, divine health ... are yours through the **provision** of Messiah by His atonement on the cross stake ("And with his stripes we are healed."), and the **promises** of God in His Word.

10

Life and **health** are yours according to the promise of God in Proverbs 4:20-22. If you have read my teachings on healing and health you know that I am NOT against doctors or seeking medical help. However, make sure God wants you to go to the doctor or to seek medical help.

Pray first, and ask God what he wants you to do. He may want to heal you instantly (or, over a period of time) without medical help.

The question is: **"Whose word will you take?"** The word of a doctor, a friend, or the Word of God? God does NOT lie, and He promises healing and health to you if you fulfill the conditions.

SCRIPTURES FOR HEALING

The Word of God builds faith for healing, is a channel for healing, a repository for healing, and an instrument for healing. Listen to it, read it, keep it in your heart. It is LIFE and HEALTH to your whole body.

There is nothing like G-d's Word.

> It builds **faith** for healing.
> It is a **channel** for healing.
> It is a **repository** of healing.
> It is an **instrument** of healing.

G-d's Word heals!

*"My son, attend to my words. Turn your ear to my sayings. Let them not depart from your eyes. Keep them in the midst of your heart. For they are **life** to those who find them, And **health** to their **whole body**."* (Proverbs 4:20-22)

I've listed several verses below from G-d's Word to help you in your healing. Read these scriptures aloud and realize **it is God talking to you through His Promises**.

■ Torah: Exodus 15:26
"If thou wilt diligently hearken to the voice of the LORD your God, and will do that which is right in his sight, and will give ear to his commandments, and keep all his statutes, I will put none of these diseases upon you, which I have brought upon the Egyptians: for I am the LORD that heals you."

■ Psalm 103:2-5
"Bless the LORD, O my soul, and forget not all his benefits: Who forgives all your iniquities; who heals all thy diseases;Who redeems your life from destruction; who crowns you with loving kindness and tender mercies; Who satisfies your mouth with good things; so that your youth is renewed like the eagle's."

■ Psalm 91:3, 5-6, 10
"For he will deliver you from the snare of the fowler, And from the deadly pestilence. You shall not be afraid of the terror by night, nor of

12

the arrow (weapon) that flies by day; Nor of the plague or disease that walks in darkness, nor of the destruction that wastes at noonday. No evil shall happen to you, neither shall any plague come near your dwelling."

■ Exodus 23:25
"And you shall serve the LORD your God, and he shall bless your bread, and your water; and I will take sickness away from the midst of you."

■ Psalm 41:4
"I said, LORD, be merciful unto me: heal my soul; for I have sinned against thee."

■ Jeremiah 33:6
"Behold, I will bring it health and cure, and I will cure them, and will reveal unto them the abundance of peace and truth."

■ Isaiah 53:5
"But he was wounded for our transgressions, he was bruised for our iniquities: the chastisement of our peace was upon him; and with his stripes we are healed."

■ 1 Peter 2:24
"Who his own self bare our sins in his own body on the tree, that we, being dead to sins, should live unto righteousness: by whose stripes you were healed."

■ 3 John 2

13

"Beloved, I wish above all things that you may prosper and be in health, even as your soul prospers."

- Psalm 107:20
"He sent his word, and healed them, and delivered them from their destructions."

- Mattiyahu (Matthew) 9:35
"And Jesus went about all the cities and villages, teaching in their synagogues, and preaching the gospel of the kingdom, and healing every sickness and every disease among the people."

- Psalm 30:2
"O LORD my God, I cried unto you, and you have healed me."

- Jeremiah 17:14
"Heal me, O LORD, and I will be healed; save me, and I will be saved: for you are my praise."

Call on Him today, my friend, and He will heal you and save you.

How to be Healed by the Laying on of Hands

The name of Yeshua (Jesus) the Messiah gives

you the **authority** and the **power** to command healing of sickness. In His Name lay hands on the sick, and they will recover.

Jesus healed the separation between G-d and man through his work FOR US, and therefore ended Satan's dominion over ALL who would trust in Christ! "For this purpose the Son of God was manifested, that he might DESTROY the works of the devil." (1 John 3:8)

Jesus "carried" sickness, sin, disease, poverty, and oppression—the works of the devil (Satan) – FOR YOU. Now you don't have to carry them any longer. They do NOT belong to the believer in Christ! WHAT JESUS DID FOR YOU ... YOU DON'T HAVE TO DO!

Now that you know that physical and mental healing belong to the believer in Christ – as much as spiritual healing – you need to know how to obtain it: HOW TO BE HEALED! There are several TOOLS, or ways, **to obtain AND to minister** Christ's healing power. They are listed below:

    THE WORD OF GOD
    LAYING ON OF HANDS
    HOLY COMMUNION
    ANOINTING WITH OIL
    PRAYER & PROPER MENTAL ATTITUDE

In the last chapter we discussed how to be healed by **the Word of God**. In this chapter I am going to teach you how to be healed by **the laying on of hands.**

LAYING ON OF HANDS

After Jesus Christ was raised from the dead and before he went back to Heaven, he said:

"And these signs shall follow them that believe; in my name shall they cast out devils; they shall speak with new tongues...they shall lay hands on the sick, and they shall recover." (Mark 16:17-18)

Notice three things that Yeshua (Jesus) said above:

> *"In my name ..."*
> *"You shall lay hands on the sick,"*
> *"They (the sick) shall recover."*

IN MY NAME–It is **the name of Jesus the Messiah**, (the Holy One of God) which is to accompany the laying on of hands. It is THE NAME that is above every name. (Philippians 2:8-9) The NAME of Jesus Christ joins God's power to your action.

The name of Jesus identifies you: it tells "sickness" and "demons" the authority behind your action and command; it tells them you belong to and are a believer in Jesus, the One who conquered them and their master, Satan! The name of Jesus identifies you with the One

16

who CREATED the world and who BOUGHT IT BACK (after Adam's sin) with his own blood!

Use the name of Jesus with authority: as a citizen of Messiah's Kingdom. If you are in doubt, just whisper the name of Jesus for a while. "Jesus, Jesus, Jesus..." It will call God's power to the scene! If it is a case of demon affliction, speak with authority (not your authority, but Christ's) and say: "You devil, come out! I command you in the name of Jesus Christ to come out of this person!"

YOU SHALL LAY HANDS ON THE SICK – If you are a believer in Jesus, then God wants to use you to heal others. You have the privilege, as well as the responsibility, of laying hands on the sick and praying for them: whether they are Christians or non-Christians. (See Luke 4:40; Acts 28:8.)

Your hands become Christ's hands: his tool! The power of the Holy Spirit flows through your hands. You may not see it, you may not feel it...but it is POWER just the same. The devil is afraid of your touch! Because of distance, sometimes, you are not able to lay hands on the sick person. (The person you want to pray for may be in a different city.) You can then send them a "prayer cloth" to be laid on the body of the sick person.

"And God wrought special miracles by the hands of Paul: so that from his body were brought unto

the sick handkerchiefs or aprons, and the diseases departed from them, and the evil spirits went out of them." (Acts 19:11-12)

Prayer cloths are very effective! Demons (evil spirits) are cast out, sick bodies are healed, and minds are restored by using them. Pray over the cloth (lay your hands on it) in the name of Jesus Christ and ask God to send deliverance, healing, and blessing. If you need a prayer cloth, email: princehandley@gmail.com.

If you are a Christian, you have more POWER than the devil ever hoped to have! Satan is afraid of your handkerchief!!

THEY SHALL RECOVER – Forget what your mind or eyes tell you. Believe what God says. You may not see the person you pray for be healed as soon as you think you should…however, you may see them be healed instantly. The important thing is to KNOW that they will recover. (Note: In some cases the sick person may be hindering their own healing; such cases will be covered later in this book under the section: *"Prayer and Proper Mental Attitude".*)

The Holy Spirit is God's agent on earth to supply the healing power of Christ. Whether the sick person is healed instantly or over a period of time–whether they feel God's power or not– Jesus promised, "These signs shall follow them that believe…they shall lay hands on the sick, and they [the sick] shall recover." Your job is to

18

serve **by faith** in obedience to Christ's command: "You go...they shall recover." Read again Mark 16:15-18 and notice the command and the promise!

How to be Healed at Passover and Holy Communion

We should expect MIRACLES during Communion and during Passover. I received an instant MIRACLE during Passover Seder at synagogue. Great pain and misery resulting from several rare diseases I developed in Africa that could not be diagnosed medically were healed instantly.

HOLY COMMUNION AND PASSOVER

You must know that healing belongs to you. There is no need for you to depart from health. You can be healed...walk in health.. and help others to do the same.

In the last chapter we discussed HOW to be healed by THE LAYING ON OF HANDS. In this one I teach you **HOW to be healed by HOLY COMMUNION** (the Lord's Supper or Eucharist), **and** also by celebrating **PASSOVER**.

We should expect MIRACLES during the Holy Communion (the Lord's Supper) and, also, during Passover. We are celebrating what Messiah did FOR US, and he told us to do this in order to remember Him until he returns. *"For as often as you eat this bread, and drink this cup, you SHOW the Lord's death until he comes [again]."* (1 Corinthians 11:26)

The Holy Bible teaches us in 1 Corinthians 11:27-32 of the Brit Chadasha (the New Testament or Covenant) that we are to do **two things** when we come to the Lord's Supper:

Discern the Lord's body, and
Examine ourselves.

To **discern** means **to see His sacrifice for us as "distinct" from other things**. See his body (the bread) beaten—even before the cross—as the Roman soldiers whipped (or flogged) him, leaving his back bruised and **striped** with open wounds. See his head **pierced** by the crown of thorns, causing blood to flow down his face and chest. And then…see his hands and feet nailed with rough spikes to the wooden cross. All of this **for us**…and **for God**!

This is why the Pesach bread, the matzo, has pin holes and stripes. At Passover, we are celebrating deliverance from bondage in Egypt…and, also, spiritual bondage; and drink the RED WINE to commemorate the RED BLOOD Messiah shed for us as **the Lamb of**

God, without fault or blemish, who takes away the sin of the world. The early Messianic believers added this matzo bread with pin holes and stripes to the Passover. Almost all the early Messianic believers in Yeshua were Jewish.

See his blood (the cup) shed for us: sinless blood, having good credit in the bank of Heaven. Not blood which inherited sin from Adam and his race, but **blood from a miracle birth** from above: as the Spirit of G-d breathed on the womb of a virgin, creating NEW LIFE from God.

"In whom we have redemption THROUGH HIS BLOOD, the forgiveness of sins, according to the riches of his grace." (Brit Chadasha: Ephesians 1:7)

"For the life of the flesh is in the blood: and I have given it to you upon the altar to make an atonement for your souls: for it is the blood that maketh an atonement for the soul." (Torah: Leviticus 17:11)

"So Messiah was once offered to bear the sins of many." (Brit Chadasha: Hebrew 9:28)

Yeshua's body and mind bore the punishment for **our** sins...his blood paid the PRICE to redeem, or ransom, **us**. And God raised him from the dead: **Yeshua is ALIVE to save and to heal you!** Yes, miracles and healing are available in the Holy Communion and the Passover by discerning the Lord's body...seeing him and what he did for us. Isaiah Chapter 53 in the Tanakh tells us:

- He bore **our** sicknesses and diseases.
- He carried (away) **our** pains.
- He was wounded and bruised for **our** sin.
- The LORD laid on him the sin of **us all**.
- And with his *stripes* **WE ARE HEALED.**

Healing by Anointing with Oil

You can be healed by the elders of the synagogue or church anointing you with oil in The Name of the LORD. There are hindrances to healing that sometimes must be dealt with and we discuss them in this chapter.

ANOINTING WITH OIL

In the Holy Bible, anointing with oil is representative of the ministry of the Ruach Elohim...the Spirit of G-d. Oil is a "type": it represents the Holy Spirit. In James 5:14-15 in the Brit Chadasha (New Testament) we read:

"Is any sick among you? Let him call for the elders of the church; and let them pray over him, anointing him with oil in the name of the Lord.

And the prayer of faith shall save the sick, and the Lord shall raise him up; and if he have committed sins, they shall be forgiven him."

It is the name, Yeshua HaMashiach (Jesus the Anointed One) accompanied by the anointing with oil and the prayer of faith that will bring your healing.

There is another type of anointing with oil which may be referred to as "evangelistic" anointing. It is just as much a part of evangelistic ministry as preaching, or teaching, or winning people to Messiah. It does NOT require the sick person to "call" for the elders of the synagogue church; nor is it only for Messianic believers.

Mark 6:12-13 tells us:

"And they went out, and preached that men should repent. And they cast out many devils, and ANOINTED WITH OIL many that were sick, and healed them."

Carry a bottle of anointing oil with you at all times, ready for use. Pray over the oil. Let God use you to heal others.

Healing Through Proper Mental Attitude

Satan is a destroyer who causes sickness and disease. God is a healer, and God calls sickness: "**captivity**. " The devil came "to steal from you, to kill you, and to destory you," but Yeshua (Jesus) came to bring you LIFE ... and life more abundantly. " Learn HOW Job – who lost everything he had, including his health – was healed.

PRAYER AND PROPER MENTAL ATTITUDE

Your mind – and therefore your body – can be abused by many things. At times there are hindrances to healing: things or conditions that are causing the sickness or affliction, and that must be dealt with before healing can take place permanently. Things such as:

- Unforgiveness, bitterness, or resentment (Mark 11:25-26)
- Envy and strife (James 3:16)
- Improper food, rest, sunshine, or exercise (Isaiah 30:15)
- Speaking evil of, or causing harm to, God's ministers (1 Samuel 26:9)

- Involvement in the occult or in witchcraft (Deuteronomy 18:10-12)
- Association with religious cults (1 John 4:1-3/1 John 5:20)

Whether sickness is caused by disobeying God through an unforgiving spirit, strife, or resentment...involvement in the occult...or association with religious cults...**Yeshua ha Meshiach (Jesus the Anointed One) is the answer!**

Through prayer we can come to God and ask Him to **forgive** us of all these things; we can also ask Him to **deliver** us, if necessary! 1 Yochanan (John) 1:9 says, *"If we confess our sins, he is faithful and just to forgive us our sins, and to cleanse us from all unrighteousness."* In Psalm 50:15 we read, *"Call upon me in the day of trouble: I will deliver you, and you shall glorify me."*

IMPORTANCE OF PROPER MENTAL ATTITUDE

We see the importance of proper mental attitude in the life of Job. Job was afflicted by Satan with sore boils from his feet to his head. Also, the devil destroyed Job's wealth and killed his seven sons and three daughters. Job's experience was a rare, "once-in-the-Bible" case. It was allowed by God to prove that a certain man ("greatest of all the men in the east") would not curse God even if he lost everything, including his health.

It shows that **Satan is a "destroyer," who causes sickness and disease**. It shows that **God is a "healer," and that God calls sickness "captivity."** Job was a just man; even God said so. His experience presents a question that many people ask: **"Why?" Notice seven keys (these are important):**

1. Job's case was unique; it was NOT an example! Don't use it as an excuse to be sick.

2. Satan accused Job of serving God only because of God's blessing, protection, and help.

3. Satan is the one, the Bible says, who STOLE Job's health, KILLED his children, and DESTROYED his property. (Job, Chapters 1 and 2; John 10:10)

4. Job proved faithful in trial. Job did not sin with his lips or charge God foolishly. (Job 1:22 and 2:10)

5. The Bible calls Job's sickness and loss "captivity." (Job 42:10). Yeshua said, "If the Son shall make you free, you shall be free indeed." (John 8:36)

6. Job was healed! Because of proper mental attitude, Job prayed for his friends (who were not real friends); this was when God delivered Job. (Job 42:10)

7. "The Lord gave Job twice as much as he had before." "The Lord blessed the latter end of Job more than his beginning." (Job 42:10-12)

Even though Job lived on the other side of the cross-stake (**before** Messiah's atonement for us)—not having the advantages of Messiah's work and authority over Satan as we do—he was still healed through prayer and proper mental attitude. A **proper mental attitude** will cause you to have an instinctive reaction to sickness and ill-health: you will **refuse** it ... knowing it does not belong to you.

You will speak to sickness, saying, "Sickness, I resist you in the name of Yeshua ha Meshiach (Jesus the Anointed One) by whose stripes I am healed."

Notice two things. You resisted the sickness by:

1. Speaking to it, and
2. Using scripture (speaking the Word of God).

The Holy Bible says in James 4:7 (Brit Chadasha), "Resist the devil, and he will flee from you." In Mattiyahu (Matthew) 4:11, we see

27

how Yeshua resisted Satan. He did it the same way you are to do it: with the Word of God. Each time Yeshua spoke to the devil, Yeshua said, "It is written ..."

It's interesting to note that each time Yeshua quoted the word of God to Satan it was from the Torah in the Book of Deuteronomy. This is the first book that was attacked in the late 1800's by so called higher criticism questioning its textual integrity. Satan hates the Book of Deuteronomy, as he does the Torah...and ALL of G-d's Holy Word.

Proper nutrition, rest, sunshine, and exercise are all beneficial to a proper mental attitude and maintenance of good health. Scriptural fasting and honoring the LORD's Day or Sabbath contribute, also, to a proper mental attitude; and are laws of G-d with built-in bonuses of health and blessing. Read Isaiah Chapter 58 in the Tanakh.

Isaiah the Prophet told 750 years before his birth how Messiah would come and be the sacrificed Lamb of God, and by whose stripes on the cross stake we would be healed. (Tanakh: Isaiah Chapter 53)

You can be healed NOW. If you want to meet the Healer, Jesus, the Anointed One, **NOW** is the time! Invite G-d's Son, Yeshua, to come into your life by praying the prayer below:

"Lord Yeshua (Jesus), I know that you are The Great Physician. You loved me enough to shed your sinless blood and die for me on the cross stake that I might be healed. I know you are alive. Please forgive my sins, come into my life, and be my Messiah. Help me to live for you, and take me to Heaven when I die."

If you prayed that prayer and meant it, then you have **eternal life and your sins are ALL forgiven**. You have been healed in your spirit. Know that God has heard and answered your prayer! The Bible says, ***"Whoever shall call upon the name of the Lord shall be saved."*** [Romans 10:13.] Notice, God did NOT say "**may** be saved" or "**might** be saved" or "**probably** will be saved," but his promise is: **"Whoever will call ... WILL BE saved!"**

Now that YOU know HOW to be healed ... YOU go bring healing to OTHERS.

Welcome to an exciting life! Live it with excellence!

Your friend,

Prince Handley

P.S. – See the following pages for other helps.

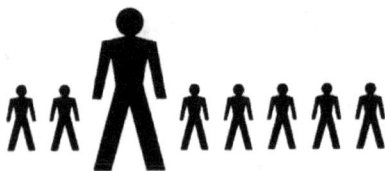

LIVE A LIFE OF EXCELLENCE

Email prayer requests and praise reports to:
princehandley@gmail.com

For a complete work on health and healing:
Health and Healing Complete Guide to Wholeness
by Prince Handley

UNIVERSITY OF EXCELLENCE PRESS

See next page for **Other Books** by Prince Handley

OTHER BOOKS BY PRINCE HANDLEY

- Map of the End Times
- How to Do Great Works
- Flow Chart of Revelation
- Action Keys for Success
- Health and Healing Complete Guide to Wholeness
- Prophetic Calendar for Israel & the Nations: To 2023
- Healing Deliverance
- How to Receive God's Power with Gifts of the Spirit
- Healing for Mental and Physical Abuse
- Victory Over Opposition and Resistance
- Healing of Emotional Wounds
- How to Be Healed and Live in Divine Health
- Healing from Fear, Shame and Anger
- How to Receive Healing and Bring Healing to Others
- New Global Strategy: Enabling Missions
- The Art of Christian Warfare
- Success Cycles and Secrets
- New Testament Bible Studies (A Study Manual)
- Babylon the Bitch: Enemy of Israel

AVAILABLE AT AMAZON AND OTHER BOOK STORES

For recent updates, go to:
www.marketplaceworld.com

UNIVERSITY OF EXCELLENCE PRESS

www.ingramcontent.com/pod-product-compliance
Lightning Source LLC
Chambersburg PA
CBHW060707280326
41933CB00012B/2334